Paleo in Maine

A Local Resource Guide for the Modern Hunter Gatherer

David Bidler

Photos of the author taken by Jes Lynch of Poetic Moments Photography. Contact Jes at poeticmoments@gmail.com.
Front cover photos from left to right are Keirsten Murphy, Gabe Garcia, and garden photo courtesy of Gabe Garcia.
All photographs in this book are used with permission.
Cover and interior design by Blaine Moore.

First Printed Edition, December 2012
Second Printed Edition, March 2013

Printed in the United States of America
Print ISBN-10: 1480164240
Print ISBN-13: 978-1480164246

Published by David Bidler
Web: www.paleoinmaine.com
Email: david@whybestrong.com

"The Paleo Diet is based on the simple understanding that the best human diet is the one to which we are best genetically adapted."
**Loren Cordain P.H.D-
author of the Paleo Diet.**

"The contemporary Paleolithic diet consists mainly of meat, fish, vegetables, fruit, roots, and nuts, and excludes grains, legumes, dairy products, salt, refined sugar, and processed oils."
The Paleo Table- Pam King

"If man made it, don't eat it."
Jack LaLane

Table of Contents

Acknowledgements

This book is dedicated to my daughters, Amella and Nikyla. My every day inspiration.

Thank you to Vanessa Antonio for her endless support, Blaine Moore for going above and beyond, and Jes Lynch for her love. I would also like to thank each and every person who has lent their spirit to this project. I am proud, grateful, and humbled to be part of such an incredible community of people.

From the heart,

David

Introduction

Paleo, a way of eating resembling that of our ancestors more than our current industrial food system, has evolved into more than a diet. It has come to represent a cultural shift in the ways that we eat, exercise, play, and live.

Referring to the Paleolithic era, the period pre-dating modern agriculture, the Paleo diet itself is a simple one. It is based on eating real foods, those which occur naturally on the earth and have been available to us for thousands of years.

The good news is that the nutrient dense foods of our ancestors are readily available. We only have to choose to eat them.

As one of many people who have embraced the future of human health by looking towards our Paleolithic past, I set out to create this simple guide to a simple way of eating.

This book is not intended to provide a complete overview of the Paleo lifestyle. Instead, it is a resource for the modern hunter-gatherer to navigate the resources available to us in our home state of Maine.

Happy hunting!
David

Local Flavor: Meeting Your "Paleo" Needs in the Modern Marketplace

The basic Paleo Diet consists of lean meats, poultry and seafood, fresh vegetables, and seasonal fruits. These simple ingredients make modern hunting and gathering a much easier task than that which our ancestors faced. However, finding snacks without refined sugars, meat without nitrates or added growth hormones, and gluten free products in a wheat dominated food system can be a challenge. Here are some tips for foraging in the modern marketplace.

1. **Hunt and Gather:** We live in a state with a wide variety of game, seasonal fruits and veggies, and a seafood population renowned throughout the world. Hunting, fishing, planting vegetables, and picking fruit are some of the most satisfying ways to stay connected to our food. Throughout this book you will find information on obtaining a hunting or fishing license, identifying medicinal herbs, and finding seasonally available "freebies" such as blueberries, morel mushrooms, and maple syrup.

2. **Support your local farmer, fisherman, or natural marketplace:** Eating locally is important to the biological needs of our bodies as well as the sustainability of our communities. Get to know your farmer. Introduce yourself to the owner of your local market. Identify the individuals who make healthy food accessible to your community and strike up a conversation!

3. **Circle the supermarket:** Shopping the perimeter of your local supermarket is a good way to avoid many canned, processed, and pre-packaged products in favor of fresh, natural food.

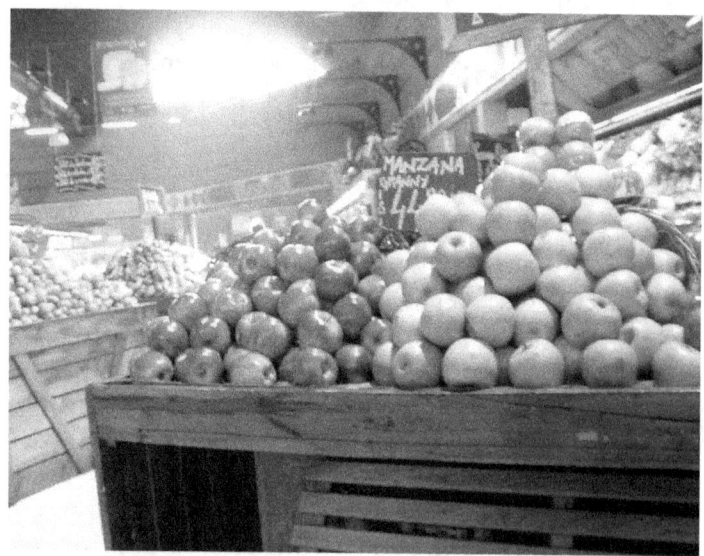

Interview with Toby Tarpinian: Owner of Morning Glory Natural Foods

Morning Glory Natural Foods has been a staple of downtown Brunswick for over 30 years. What factors do you attribute to the long term success of the business?

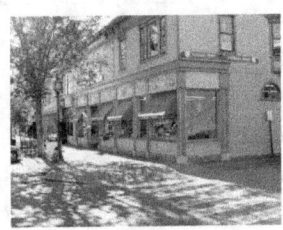

I really think that it comes down to being a family owned local business with competitive prices. When my mom opened up the store 31 years ago, the sale of natural foods and products was truly a fringe market. I remember her trying to get a bank loan for what was viewed at the time as a quirky and expensive specialty store. I don't think that she brought home a dime for the first seven years, but she worked hard to grow the business and meet the evolving needs of her customers and eventually it paid off.

I think that one of my mom's greatest strengths was smart purchasing which allows us to pass on our volume discount to our customers. That and her ability to innovate while staying responsive to her customers helped to develop the business throughout those early years.

By the time that I finished college and prepared to take over the day to day operations here at Morning Glory, the natural foods movement had grown significantly. I contribute a lot of this growth to people like my mom and others who were ahead the curve with their vision for distributing healthy, locally sourced food in the community. I think that another factor in our success is our focus on buying local.

30% of our store is made up of local products and we would take a local product at a higher price over a less expensive out-of-state option any day.

What products can you find on the shelves of Morning Glory that you might not find at some of the national retailers such as Whole Foods and Trader Joe's?

Meats, dairy, and produce directly from Maine farms. Many of the larger nationwide chains purchase their products from similarly large national distributors. Alternatively, our products come directly from the hands of farmers throughout the state. Items such as organic meats and cheeses, honey, maple syrup, homemade jams and spreads, and local organic coffee are delivered to us daily by the Crown of Maine Organic Cooperative, a local distributor of Maine-made products. The few large retailers that carry these items do so at a 100% mark-up while our commitment to local purchasing allows us to buy these products at volume and pass along those savings to the customer.

Morning Glory has an impressive selection of free-range meats and poultry from farms throughout the state, much of which might otherwise be inaccessible to local residents. What are some of the most sought after items and where do they come from?

Local meat is the most sought after item of all. The grass fed beef and sausages from A Wee Bit Farm in Orland are particularly popular as are the products from Eastern River Cattle based in Dresden, Maine.

Raw milk is another product that has been increasingly popular. Here in Maine, a farmer can go out in the morning to milk his cow, put the milk in a bucket, and take it over to our store to sell. While many states impose varying levels of restriction on raw milk consumption or ban its sale altogether, consumers in Maine can research the proposed health benefits of raw milk and decide for themselves if they want to drink it.

I know that milk isn't included in most interpretations of the Paleo diet but our customers who do consume dairy products have responded to the opportunity to purchase milk directly from Maine dairy farms that hasn't been put through the various ringers of pasteurization.

Aside from that, it is our selection of gluten free products that customers are really responding to. We have also seen a spike in the sales of bulk nuts and coconut products over recent months.

How have the dietary preferences of your customers changed over the past three decades?

In the beginning it was natural as opposed to organic, there was a large demand for dairy and meat alternatives, and our customer base consisted mainly of individuals on alternative diets. Now, more and more people are concerned over whether their food has been sprayed with one chemical or another or whether their meat was raised free-range and grass-fed. People are increasingly attracted to foods in their raw form such as nuts, seeds, and minimally processed products with little to nothing done to them. In general, customers are looking towards products with as few ingredients as possible.

A heightened interest in what we eat and how it affects our bodies has created an increased demand for the products of Maine farmers and food distributors. At the same time we've seen the natural food aisles of many major retailers expand and an influx of seemingly healthy but far from local products hit the shelves. Can you share some thoughts on the future of food in Maine and how we as consumers can help to shape it?

I'm thankful to say that business at Morning Glory has continued to grow every year. Even with the economy, people who have never walked into a natural food store are crossing the threshold as information on the relationship between diet and health becomes more readily available.

Documentaries on topics such as genetically modified foods or conventional methods of food production have raised an unprecedented level of awareness about what we eat and where it comes from. Many of our newer customers have come into the store after watching a film that inspired them to eat better while others come in based on the suggestions of their doctors, many of whom are becoming increasingly aware of the connection between health and nutrition and passing this information along to their patients.

So to answer the question directly, I think that information and education are the most important tools that we can use to shape the future of food in Maine. I feel that having knowledgeable employees to guide customers through the process of selecting healthy natural foods while answering their questions is extremely important.

For example, here at Morning Glory we have an in-store nutritionist who can help guide customers through a shopping experience that may be largely unfamiliar to them. Most importantly, if we hope to sustain this movement, we have to educate ourselves and each other on the benefits of buying locally.

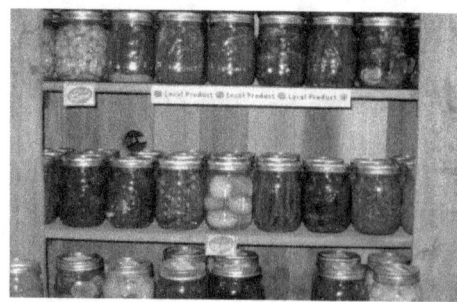

Visit Morning Glory Natural Foods at 60 Maine Street in Brunswick or go to www.moglonf.com for more information.

Dining Out: A Survivors Guide

While there are no "Paleo" specific restaurants in our state, keep in mind that Paleo involves a very simple approach to eating which can be easily applied when dining out. A big fresh salad with a lean cut of steak is a perfect Paleo meal providing that the ingredients are fresh and meet your personal quality standards.

The questions below are ones that any quality restaurant should be able to answer, and their ability to do so may serve as a marker of whether or not to keep it in your regular restaurant rotation. Here are some good questions for your local restaurant, owner, chef, or server:

What to ask before you order:

- What farms do you get your meat, poultry, and produce from?
- What oils do you use to prepare your food?
- Do you offer gluten-free menu options?
- Do you use bread crumbs or other gluten containing products as fillers in any of your recipes?
- What additional measures do you take to eliminate cross-contamination of gluten?

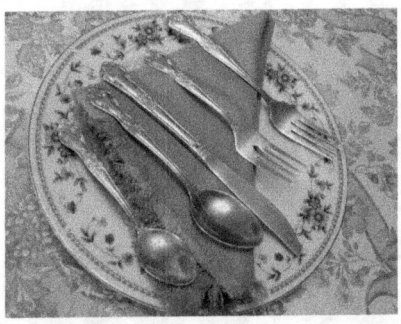

Interview with Jonah Fertig: Owner of Local Sprouts Cooperative

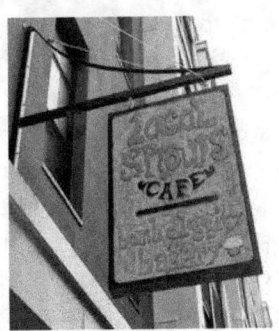

Since opening its doors in 2009 Local Sprouts has become a staple of downtown Portland. How did the business grow from a concept into the vibrant community space that it is today?

Local Sprouts took many hands and a lot of community support to grow from an idea that started 5 years ago into a worker cooperative that today has 25 worker-owners and provides local and organic food through our Café and catering services, as well as our education and outreach programs.

All along the way we have reached out to our community and received support through time, skills, money, ideas and more. In turn, Local Sprouts has supported our community through providing healthy food, supporting local farmers, creating a welcoming and comfortable space for the community, and supporting people with their visions for creating cooperative businesses and projects.

Local Sprouts is Portland's first Community Supported Café. How does this business model work and why is it beneficial to both the customer and the owner?

We received the majority of our start-up funds through individual loans from friends and families in our community. We also had many people that became members of our Community Supported Kitchen and have given money up front. In our renovation process we had close to 200 people that helped to create the space.

This has benefited Local Sprouts through providing a strong base of support and receiving funds from people that support our mission and didn't charge us lots of interest.

It has also been beneficial to the customers in creating a sense of belonging to something that is creating good in the community. Through supporting Local Sprouts, people are supporting creating cooperative jobs, supporting local farms, supporting local food education and organizing, and creating a positive impact on their community.

Local Sprouts has achieved remarkable success with its values of cooperative ownership, locally supported agriculture, and community development intact. What advice would you give to socially conscious upstarts seeking to balance these principles with the realities of business ownership?

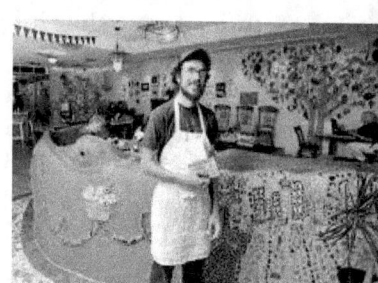

Jonah Fertig:
Worker-Owner at Local Sprouts

It is really important to learn business skills and to balance ideals with business efficiency. If your business fails, then your ideals and values will go down with it.

We do business differently, but there are many things that are similar in starting up any small business. It is important to learn those business skills and get the support from people in the business development community so that you can create a solid business plan and get a strong financial structure in place.

When you are approaching business from an ethical and cooperative perspective, you will be constantly questioning and evaluating the assumptions of conventional business.

So there is a continual balancing act but if done well and with community support it can be successful.

Visit Local Sprouts Café at 649 Congress Street in Portland or go to www.localsproutscooperative.com for more information.

Paleo-Goodies: Local Distributors of Paleo-Friendly Products

Harvest Time Natural Foods
171 Capitol St. Suite 1
Augusta, ME
207-623-8700

Belfast Coop Store
123 High St.
Belfast, ME
207-338-2532
www.belfastcoop.com

New Morning Natural Foods
230 Main St.
Biddeford, ME
207-282-1434

Morning Dew Natural Foods
19 Sandy Creek Rd.
Bridgton, ME
207-647-4003
www.morningdewnatural.com

Nature's Choice
87 Elm St.
Camden, ME
207-236-8280

Natural Living Center
209 Longview Dr.
Bangor, ME
207-990-2646
www.naturallivingcenter.net

Good Food Store
212 Mayville Rd.
Bethel, ME
207-824-3754
www.goodfoodbethel.com

Blue Hill Co-Op Inc.
Green's Hill Plaza
Blue Hill, ME

Morning Glory Natural Foods
60 Maine St.
Brunswick, ME
207-729-0546
www.moglonf.com

Rising Tide Natural Foods Coop
15 Coastal Market Dr.
Damariscotta, ME
207-563-5556
www.risingtide.coop

Bob's Farm Home & Garden
15 Lincoln
Dover-Foxcroft, ME
207-564-2581

Better Living Center
181 Front St.
Farmington, ME
207-778-6018

New Morning Natural Foods
3 York St.
Kennebunk, ME
207-985-6774
www.newmorningnaturalfoods.com

Earth's Bounty
57 Fleming St.
Lincoln, ME
207-794-8266

Fare Share Market
443 Main St.
Norway, ME
207-743-9044

Whole Foods
127 Marginal Way
Portland, ME
Phone: 207-774-7711

John Edwards Market Inc
158 Main St.
Ellsworth, ME
207-667-9377
www.johnedwardsmarket.com

Royal River Natural Foods
443 US Route 1
Freeport, ME
207-865-0046
Website: www.rrnf.com

Center For Healthy Living
118 Old Post Rd.
Kittery, ME
207-439-1988
www.cfhl.com

Endless Herbs & Natural Foods
67 Moosehead Trail
Newport, ME
207-368-7743

The Store/Ampersand
22 Mill St.
Orono, ME
207-866-4592

Good Tern Natural Foods Store
750 Main St.
Rockland, ME
207-594-8822
www.goodtern.com

Fresh Off The Farm
495 Commercial St.
Rockport, ME
207-236-3260

Red Hill Natural Foods
228 Waldo St.
Rumford, ME
207-369-9141

Lois's Natural Market
152 US Route 1
Scarborough, ME
207-885-0602
www.loisnatural.com

Nezinscot Farm
284 Turner Center Rd.
Turner, ME
Phone: 207-225-3231
www.nezinscotfarm.com

Sheepscot General Store
98 Townhouse Rd.
Whitefield, ME
207-549-5185
www.sheepscotgeneral.com

Neighborhood Healthy & Herbs
23 Main St.
Saco, ME
207-286-8633

Spice Of Life
432 Madison Ave
Skowhegan, ME
Phone: 207-474-8216

Uncle Dean's Groceries
80 Grove St.
Waterville, ME
207-873-6231

Farms and Markets

The website of the Maine Organic Farmers and Gardeners Association (MOFGA) maintains an excellent listing of all the farms and farmers markets in Maine.

Visit their website to find one near you: www.mofga.com

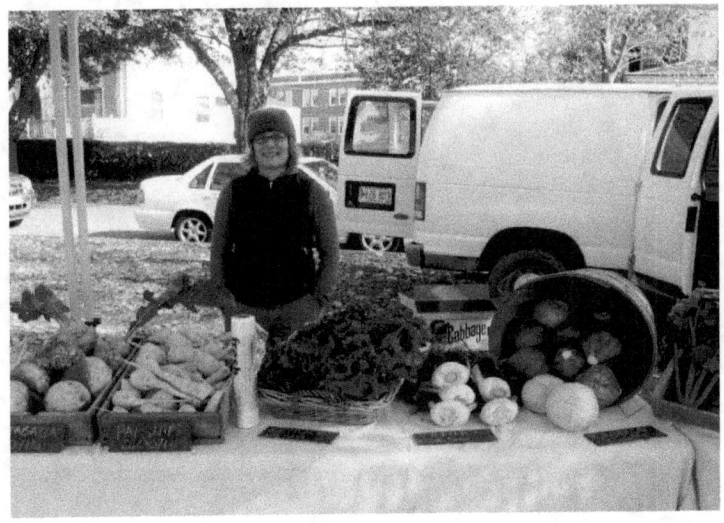

Sarah Trask of Small Wonders Organics at the Brunswick farmers market

Interview with Ralph Caldwell: Owner of Caldwell Farms

The agricultural industry has seen some major changes since the early 1940's when your parents first started the farm. What did a typical day on the farm look like when you were a child? How does it look now, today, for your children?

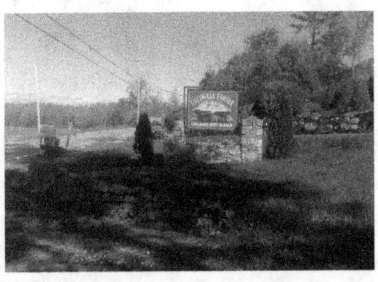

We had started out with 5 cows to milk in the mid 1940's. My mother and father worked in the woods, my father cut logs and pulp, my mother twitched the wood with horses and we came along as kids.

I never had a babysitter in my life! We didn't go anywhere, we just farmed.

It was a way of life. Everything was done by hand in that era, there were no hydraulics. There were no hydraulic pumps, no hydraulic cylinders, and no loaders. It's changed now to where almost nothing is done by hand; it's all done by machine.

As far as how the day looks for me and my children nowadays, well, we start milking at 2 am. My daughter and myself and my oldest grandson will work about 80 hours in a week but we like what we do, and we like where we do it, and we like who we do it with.

Caldwell Farms operated as a dairy farm for nearly 50 years before entering into organic and natural beef

production. What led to this decision, how has it impacted your business, and which product do you see leading Caldwell into the future?

As you say, we were straight dairy until 1999. In the late 1990's we had made up our minds that we probably were going to exit the dairy industry. The margins were very slim.

We were milking 3 times a day and had the second highest herd average in the state of Maine, but the Southwest can raise milk for about 30% less than we can. A cousin of mine went in with Organic Valley in 1997 and they were trying to grow the organic milk industry and were paying twice as much as the conventional alternative.

We did well from 1999 through 2005 until ethanol came along. Ethanol has been the single greatest challenge to ever hit animal agriculture. It took the cost of caring for and raising animals to a level that you pretty much just can't get around.

Corn is everything in the diet of the world and everything else is tied to it. Corn went from $2 a bushel to $6 a bushel in a year and a half. That year the drought hit in the southwest and corn went to $8.50. Organic corn rose to $14 a bushel. I was paying $5 for it a year ago. The price of milk is thirty dollars a hundred and it has been for several years. We were just being killed and this is what led us to branch out into the beef industry.

With an increasing demand for grass-fed beef, do you have any plans to eliminate the transitional feed and non-GMO grains that you use and make a move in this direction?

I think that it is another niche market. There is nothing wrong with the concept; the issue is that cattle need approximately 75 therms of net energy to maintain themselves year-round.

Grass, even wicked good grass, has 62-63 therms, and in cold weather they can't get energy enough to maintain their weight.

Now, their diet doesn't have to be as high in energy in the summertime as it does in the wintertime. In climates like South America or Central America, where it's summer all year long, it's not a bad concept. In the state of Maine there are some issues that I won't subject my cattle to and that's why I don't have grass fed beef. A cow can do pretty good on grass once they've matured and gotten their structure built. If they would let me feed them until they were 13-14 months old I think it would be a good idea but that's not allowed.

As the public becomes more conscious of what they're eating and where it comes from, the power of big agribusiness corporations is on the rise as well. What are some of the new opportunities as well as new challenges facing Maine farmers given the heightened interest in their products along with the heightened competition in the market?

We have the advantage of closeness to the consumer. We have a segment of the population that wants to know where their food is coming from and how it's raised.

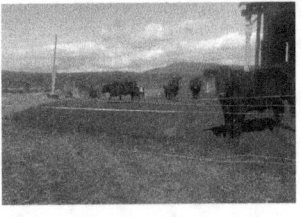

We also have a segment of the population that is lactose intolerant that can drink our milk. The enzymes to process milk are in the milk. When you cook it, you kill it. It doesn't mean that you can't drink milk; it means that you can't drink pasteurized milk. Raw milk works.

Our customers are well educated, are aware of the fact that you are what you eat, and feel like some agriculture in the state of Maine would be a nice thing.

As far as the products that will lead Caldwell Farms into the future, I really feel that our frozen dinner line will be our salvation to continuing to be in business. The last crop that is planted on a dairy farm is houses and we're borderline. If it was only the dairy business we'd be planting houses. There are no local, organic, and gluten-free frozen dinners available right now and I think that there's a market for it. I truly believe that if we've got a salvation, that's it.

Visit www.caldwellfarmsmaine.com or call 207-225-3871 for more info.

Hunt and Gather: A Beginners Guide to Hunting, Fishing and Foraging in Maine

From blueberries, cranberries, and maple syrup to sea vegetables, shellfish, and wild morel mushrooms, a number of seasonal "freebies" can be found by foraging through the forest or digging along Maine's coast.

One of the best resources on local foraging exists on the website of the United States Department of Agriculture Forest Service at www.fs.fed.us. This site includes a comprehensive handbook on plant identification as well as information on the cultural and ecological landscape of northern Maine and its Canadian neighbors through the non-timber forest products that grow in our region and the people who gather and depend on them.

Visit www.fs.fed.us for more information.

Maine Primitive Skills School hosts a comprehensive series of educational classes and interactive workshops on topics such as native awareness, plant identification, and tracking, as well as wilderness survival.

Visit www.primitiveskills.com for more info for more information.

The Maine Department of Inland Fisheries is an excellent resource on hunting and fishing for beginners. Their website includes detailed information on licensing, legal regulations, and educational courses to get you started.

Visit www.maine.gov/ifw/ or call 207-287-8000 for more information.

Paleo Fitness

As hunters and gatherers, our ability to move heavy objects out of our paths, sprint to chase our prey, and travel for long periods of time determined our ability to survive. These periods of exertion were ideally followed by periods of rest, and together they represent a blueprint for physical fitness which our genes best respond to.

"Move frequently at a slow pace, lift heavy things, sprint once in a while."

Mark Sisson, author of the Primal Blueprint and the popular nutrition blog Mark's Daily Apple

Today, more and more of us are rejecting the conventional gym model and staying fit by integrating fun, spontaneity, and community into our workouts. Explosive and dynamic movements such as kettle bell swings are replacing endless dumbbell curls and hours on the treadmill.

Programs such as CrossFit, which are based on constantly varied and high intensity workouts performed in a group setting, are replacing the chronic cardio sessions of the past. Add to this the opportunity to learn and practice new skills such as martial arts or yoga and you have the foundation for a lifestyle from which a healthy and strong body comes naturally.

Not surprisingly, the most successful fitness programs prioritize nutrition. With a healthy diet, sound sleep, and reduced stress it doesn't take much "exercise" to stay fit, lean, and strong. Here are some local options for staying fit the paleo way:

Play Outside: Let a child loose in a field, on a beach, or along a wooded trail, and watch as their imagination transforms these common areas into places of play.

Activities such as climbing, running, and jumping come naturally to us. As a result, natural, functional fitness gains come along with them. There are many opportunities to establish increased mobility, flexibility, power, strength, and speed right in your own backyard. Here are some ideas:

Get Mobile: Bear crawls, squats, handstands, sprints, long jumps, burpees, and countless other movements can be performed wherever there is open space and an open mind. The ability to move our bodies in a variety of ways is essential to our long term mobility and there are countless options for developing these body-weight movements into creative and challenging workouts.

Try these: Pick a combination of movements (10 push-ups, 10 air squats, and a 400 meter bear crawl for example) and see how many rounds you can complete in 20 minutes!

Run Trails: Pick your favorite walking/hiking trail and pick up the speed. Maine has some spectacular running trails all across the state and hosts some of the best trail races in the country.

Here are a few of the best local trails:

Bradbury Mountain
528 Hallowell Rd.
Pownal, ME
207-688-4712
www.bradburymountain.com

Pineland Farms
15 Farm View Dr.
New Gloucester, ME
207-688-4539
www.pinelandfarms.org

The Appalachian Trail
www.appalachiantrail.org

The Eastern Trail
www.easterntrail.org

Trail Monster Running hosts weekly group runs and organizes some of the best trail races around.

Vist them out at www.trailmonsterrunning.com for more information.

Inside the "Box":
Local CrossFit Affiliates

CrossFit 321
4 Turner St.
Brunswick, ME
207-729-8200
www.crossfit321.com

CrossFit 207
1625 Maine St. #310
Sanford, ME
207-651-8529
www.crossfit207.com

CrossFit Beacon
341 Marginal Way
Portland, ME
207-619-2232
www.crossfitbeacon.com

CrossFit Camp Keyes
194 Winthrop St.
Augusta, ME
www.crossfitcampkeyes.com

Ship City CrossFit
111 Center St.
Bath, ME
www.shipcitycrossfit.com

CrossFit MF
429 Warren Ave
Portland, ME
207-619-1986
www.crossfitmf.com

CrossFit Undaunted
265 Water St.
Augusta, ME
207-514-5734
www.crossfitundaunted.com

CrossFit Casco Bay
1000 Congress St.
Portland, ME
207-699-4080
www.crossfitcascobay.com

Stone Coast CrossFit
16 Rockport Park Center Rd.
Rockport, ME
207-370-0544
www.stonecoastcrossfit.com

CrossFit Acadia
249 Bucksport Rd.
Ellsworth, ME
207-266-3726
www.crossfitacadia.com

CrossFit Bangor
615 Odlin Rd.
Bangor, ME
www.crossfitbangor.com

Mixing it Up: Mixed Martial Arts Schools in Maine

Gracie Barra Maine
424 Odin Rd.
Bangor, ME
207-947-0763
www.graciebarramaine.com

Team Irish Mixed Martial Arts
34 Abbott St.
Brewer, ME
207-433-0420
www.teamirishmma.com

Huard's Jujitsu and Karate
234 Clinton Ave
Winslow, ME
207-649-8080
www.huards.com

Foundry Brazilian Jiu Jitsu
Academy-Farmington
189 Perham St.
Farmington, ME
207-778-0485
www.foundrybjj.com

Maine Jiu Jitsu Academy
638 Wiscasset Rd.
Boothbay, ME
207-633-6552
www.mainejiujitsu.com

Foundry Brazilian Jiu Jitsu -
Rangely
25 Dallas Hill Rd.
Rangely, ME
207-864-3332
www.foundrybjj.com

MMA Athletix
101 Leeman Hgwy.
Bath, ME
207-751-8835
www.mmaathletix.com

The Academy
651 Riverside St.
Portland, ME
207-615-0060
www.theacademymaine.com

Dragon Fire Mixed Martial Arts
156 Pleasant Hill Rd.
Scarborough, ME
207-809-9223
www.Dragonfireme.com

Havoc Mixed Martial Arts
and Group Fitness
898 Main St.
Sanford, ME
207-459-9494
www.havocmma.com

Team Irish Mixed Martial Arts-
Biddeford
117 Maine St
Biddeford, ME
207-671-2168
www.teamirishmma.com

Yoga, Gymnastics, Swimming, and Dance

There are far too many fitness centers to list individually but explore your community for programs, classes, and activities that inspire you and take the personal plunge into paleo-fitness.

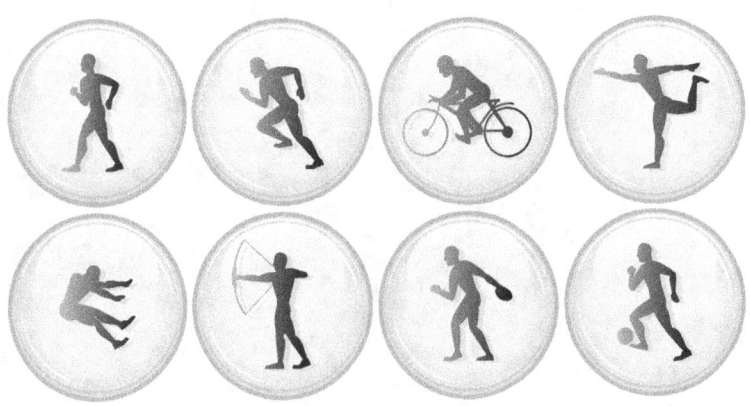

Finding Your Passion...

Passion is the key ingredient to creating a lasting lifestyle change. One of the services that I offer to my clients is individualized fitness consulting. My goal is to help others identify the markers of any quality fitness program and pursue those which spark their personal passion.

Visit www.whybestrong.com for more information.

My Diet to Keep: Paleo Tips from CrossFit Coach Gabe Garcia

First let me say that I am honored to contribute to David's work. Since the day I met him I have been inspired by his passion and drive. He is truly dedicated to educating and coaching others into healthier lifestyles.

I have had an extremely competitive spirit since I was born. As one of six kids I had to compete for anything and everything. I played soccer at an elite level through my youth and went on to play at Division 1 at Wofford College. After the end of my competitive sports career, I was nudged by my sister to try CrossFit and I was hooked from the first workout. I compete regularly in CrossFit competitions and was honored to represent CrossFit 321 at the CrossFit Games Northeast Regional in 2012.

I am also a certified Level 1 CrossFit instructor. Nutrition has always been a passion of mine and I was introduced to the Paleo Diet through CrossFit. I am currently a CrossFit coach and routinely offer nutrition coaching to my athletes.

My Paleo story began September of 2010 in Franklin, Tennessee. I took part in a Whole 30 Challenge with my member affiliate, CrossFit Talon. I had been CrossFitting for a while and definitely saw results from the exercise.

I had read some Paleo books and cut out grains, dairy, and sugar from my diet. It wasn't too big of a change from my previous diet, aside from the frequent pasta and pizza I ate previously. However, I wanted to experience what the Paleo buzz was about and see for myself if it really would improve my performance and health.

I started the challenge weighing 155 pounds with 7% body fat. In the first week I lost a little over 5 pounds and was probably at an unhealthy body fat percentage. I had to add healthy fats and make myself eat more, which was a challenge.

Once I learned what my body needed, the benefits were amazing. I felt better in almost every way: digestion, sleep, recovery from training, mood, and energy. All this was an improvement from a baseline that was pretty healthy to begin with. I also began to really taste food that was masked by sugar, salt, and other additives. It definitely was an awakening to my mind, body, and spirit.

After the challenge, I was so happy with the results that I decided Paleo would be my diet to keep.

I don't believe it worked miracles or made me super-human in any way, but it definitely made me more of a human. More than ever before, I felt an awareness of my body and how the foods I consume affect it. I was curious about how I would deal with adding non-Paleo foods back into my diet. I found that dairy was no problem, but that I really did not feel well after sugar, grains, or beans/legumes. So now I occasionally cheat with the things that don't bother me, and very rarely cheat with the things that don't make me feel my best.

Eating Paleo has been a challenge at times because my wife and 2 year old son do not follow the diet. I routinely experiment with many modifications to the diet in order to meet the demands of my training habits and goals. I also believe in experimenting with other diets that are backed by research and positive results.

I have not found a diet anywhere near as beneficial and effective as Paleo.

Here are my top 5 Tips for Paleo:

1. Make it fun by adding variety. Try new things with an open mind. You will be surprised what by what you like.
2. Have someone hold you accountable. Better yet, tell everyone around you that you are eating Paleo and they will watch closely to see if you cheat.
3. Don't worry about counting calories or pounds lost, that will take care of itself.
4. Record your results. Did you sleep longer, more soundly, and wake up feeling refreshed? Has your digestion become more regular? Do you feel more energy during the day?
5. Practice 80/20 or 90/10:
   a. Plan your cheats: if you know there is a Super Bowl party on Sunday, eat clean until then.
   b. Take advantage of your cheats and then move on without regret. If you cheat small, with one meal (a bite of cake, a little cheese), you will still feel like you are due a cheat meal.
   c. Cheat with foods that do not make you feel terrible. If grains make you gassy, you may have gluten allergies and should avoid them.

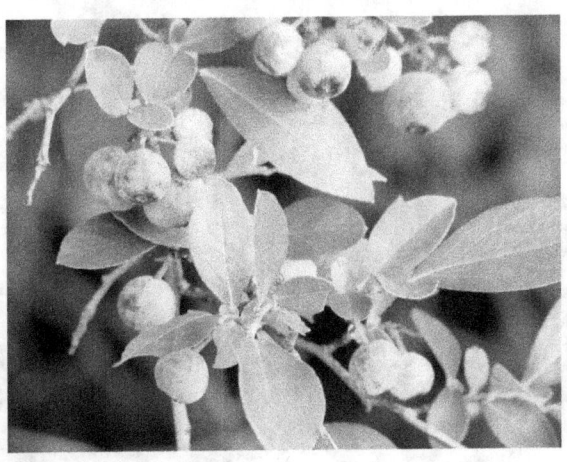

Here are my time saving methods:

1. Prepare food for the week. Use lists, menus, and batched food preparation such as chopping, mixing, etc.
2. Always have emergency ingredients and staples to fall back on.
3. Plan meals that are interchangeable and have carryover into the other meals of the week.
4. Cook in bulk and don't be afraid to freeze food you don't finish. With no preservatives, things can spoil more quickly than you may be used to. Many stews, chili, and sauces freeze well.
5. Organize recipes in a common area near the kitchen so they are available when you are cooking.
6. Learn to love your crock-pot. Anything can be cooked in it and usually tastes great.
7. Frozen vegetables are just as delicious as fresh. Well, some are at least. They are inexpensive and can be great when fresh veggies are not in season.
8. Learn to love your food processor.
9. Wing It! Free hand cooking to your tastes can be fun and fast. Learn to let go and explore.
10. Paleo-ize your non Paleo cookbooks and meals.

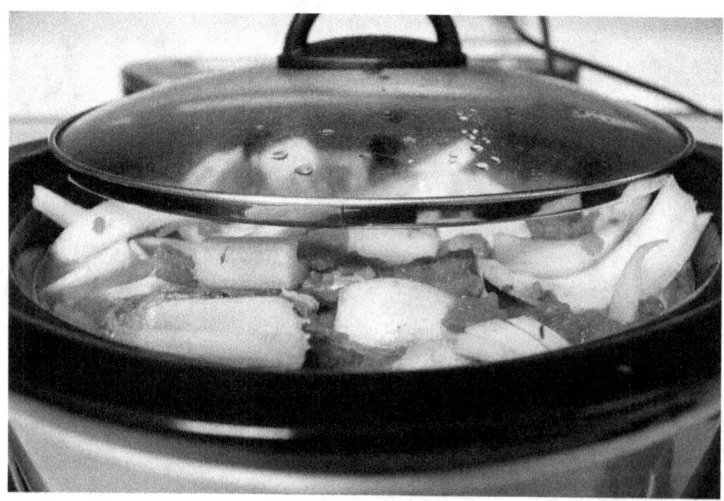

You must always have these kitchen staples on hand. If you run out, immediately stop what you are doing and restock.

1. Spices:
    a. Cayenne Pepper Powder
    b. Cinnamon
    c. Chili Powder
    d. Cumin
    e. Curry Powder
    f. Garlic Powder
    g. Onion Powder
    h. Paprika or smoked paprika
    i. Red Pepper Flakes
    j. Sea Salt/Kosher Salt
    k. Penzeys spices has a ton of great spices and many salt free spice mixtures. You can order from http://www.penzeys.com/
2. Oils and Sauces
    a. Almond oil – awesome alternative oil for salad dressings
    b. Balsamic Vinegar
    c. Coconut Oil
    d. Extra Virgin Olive Oil
    e. Hot Sauce (read your labels, I use Franks)
    f. Macadamia nut oil – great for nut butters
    g. Red wine vinegar
3. Foods
    a. Cage Free Eggs
    b. Coconut Milk – full fat in the can, no preservatives or water if possible. I use Whole Foods Brand.
    c. Nuts
    d. Avocado
    e. Boneless Skinless Chicken Breasts – stock your freezer full
    f. Lots of fresh veggies and fruit

A Day in the Life: Recipes and Sample Meal Plans by Keirsten Murphy of Keirsten's Kitchen

"Paleo, to me, is about eating modern versions of foods that we have eaten for thousands of years that are available to us in the wild today…what the human body was engineered to eat."

"Don't get hung up with the 'is this paleo' disposition, rather, ask yourself how the food that you are about to eat will nourish your body. Where does it come from? How was it made? Has it been refined or processed? Does it exist now, in nature? This is what Keirsten's Kitchen is all about. It's Paleo…ish."

from Keirsten's Kitchen

Sample meal plan:

Breakfast: Bacon, Apple, and Egg Salad- Chopped organic apple, baked bacon, and hard boiled eggs served over a bed of greens with balsamic vinaigrette or honey mustard dressing.

Lunch: Quick Paleo Lunch Wraps-Thinly sliced roast beef, fresh radishes, and mayonnaise wrapped in leaf of crisp romaine lettuce.

Dinner: Ranch Meatloaf with Garlic Fiddleheads-Grass-fed ground beef baked with chopped peppers, onions, and a little bit of dill. Covered with Keirsten's home-made ranch dressing and served alongside fresh fiddleheads sautéed in garlic.

Dessert: Coconut Cream and Berry Parfait-Fresh local berries layered with coconut milk and garnished with fresh mint.

Visit www.keirstenskitchen.com for recipes and delicious meal options.

Blueberry Pancakes:

Ingredients:

1 well-ripened banana
3 large spoonfuls of almond butter
2 eggs
2 Tbsp. thawed wild Maine blueberries, or fresh when in season
Butter for cooking

Preparation:

Mash the banana in a medium-sized mixing bowl
Mix in the egg and almond butter
Mix well
Melt butter in a frying pan over medium heat
Drop spoonfuls of the pancake batter onto the pan once butter is melted
Drop blueberries on top of pancake
(If you mix the blueberries into the batter, they may sink to the bottom of your pancakes and stick to the pan while cooking!)
When the edges of the pancake begin to have air bubbles coming up, flip the pancake and continue to cook for a few minutes on the other side. Enjoy!

Apple, Basil, Ginger Burgers:

Ingredients:

Few fresh basil leaves
1- 1/2 Tbsp. fresh ginger, chopped fine
1/2 medium apple, chopped fine
1 lb. grass-fed ground beef
*If ginger and apple are not chopped fine, the burgers will fall apart while cooking.

Preparation:

Combine all ingredients in a medium bowl
Make into burger patties
Grill or cook in frying pan to desired temperature or wellness
Enjoy over a salad, add bacon or eat with your favorite vegetables

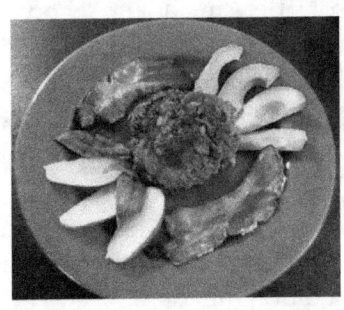

Paleo-Apple Crisp:

Ingredients:

4 Apples
Variety of nuts to equal 2 cups (this recipe used almonds, Brazil nuts and hazelnuts)
2 tsp. ground cinnamon
1tsp. ground nutmeg
1 tbsp. butter
1 tbsp. raw honey (or raw maple syrup)
2 spoonfuls almond butter

Preparation:

Chop apples into small pieces
Place in baking dish
Add 1 tbsp. butter
Add cinnamon and nutmeg
Cover and bake at 400 for 12-15 minutes
While apples are baking, chop all nuts in a food processor (Be sure not to chop to a powder- leave some nuts in larger pieces)
Add almond butter and honey, mix well. Remove apples from oven and stir
Spread almond butter mixture over the apples, one spoonful at a time
Return to the oven and bake at 400 for 10-12 minutes, or until the almond butter mixture starts to brown a bit on the top
Remove from oven and serve!

Recommended Reading

The Paleo Solution by Robb Wolf: Robb Wolf, one of the world's leading experts on Paleolithic nutrition, presents a fun and easily digestible primer for anyone interested in the Paleo diet. A recommended first-stop on the road to Paleo research and literature.

The Paleo Answer by Loren Cordain: A sequel to The Paleo Diet, University of Colorado Professor Loren Cordain's first major book on Paleolithic nutrition includes the most recent research on all things Paleo.

The Primal Blueprint by Mark Sisson: A creative and uniquely independent take on the lives of our Paleolithic ancestors. The Primal Blueprint tells the tale of human evolution through the character Grok (the archetypal primal human) and emphasizes elements such as play, leisure, and the role of relationships and community.

Everyday Paleo by Sarah Fragaso: Hands down, one of the most informative and accessible paleo books on the market. Sarah covers all of the basics of the Paleo-lifestyle and provides a ton of great recipes to get you started!

Worthwhile Websites

paleotable.com	The Paleo Table: Paleo dining made easy by writer Pam King.
marksdailyapple.com	Mark's Daily Apple: Primal Living in the Modern Word by author Mark Sisson.
robbwolf.com	Revolutionary Solutions to Modern Life: The website of Paleo pioneer Robb Wolf.
keirstenskitchen.com	Keirsten's Kitchen: A truly stand-out site from a Portland based Paleo chef. An extensive collection of recipes accompanied by a unique perspective on the Paleo lifestyle.
eatmainefoods.org	Eat Maine Foods: A networking site of the Eat Local Foods Coalition of Maine. The Eat Maine Foods website includes an interactive map listing community supported agriculture, local farm stands, specialty food stores, and organic buying clubs in your area.
eatwild.com	Eat Wild: The clearinghouse for information on pasture raised farming and grass -fed food.
on.fb.me/14wiwDP	100: Head Heart and Feet is a feature length documentary following Zak Wieluns as he runs the Vermont 100.

primitiveskills.com	The Maine Primitive Skills School is a wilderness survival school located in Augusta Maine. Their mission is to provide and preserve ancient survival skills that promote awareness and self sufficiency with an emphasis on individuals, their communities, and the environments in today's world. They host an extensive variety of educational classes which are listed on their website.
paleoparents.com	Paleo Parents: The Paleo Parents blog is about a practical and affordable approach to feeding their family real food.
paleohacks.com	Paleo Hacks: A place to ask questions about the Paleo diet, exercise, and lifestyle.
health-bent.com	Health-Bent: The website of South Carolina couple Brandon and Megan Keatly, Health-Bent is dedicated to pursuing health through food. Includes great recipes and a straightforward approach to beginning the paleo lifestyle.
chriskresser.com	Chris Kresser: Medicine for the 21st Century: Your online go-to destination for delving into common myths and misunderstandings about health and medicine.

About the Author

I am a writer, a father, and a personal fitness coach living in Portland, Maine.

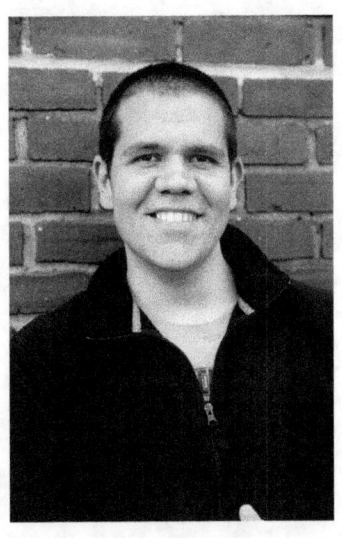

I wrote this book because I think that the way that we eat is important. What we put in our bodies determines the way that we feel, which in turn determines the way that we live. From our interactions with one another, to how we approach our goals, to the types of communities that we build, our approach to life is shaped by whether we feel healthy, strong, and confident in ourselves.

I hope that it leads to conversations about strength of body as well as strength of spirit and that it serves you well on your path towards health, wellness, and the personal goals that lie on your horizon.

Eat well, stay strong, and pass it on,
David

Visit www.whybestrong.com for more information on personal training and fitness consultation services.

Visit www.paleoinmaine.com for a listing of upcoming presentations and events.

www.ingramcontent.com/pod-product-compliance
Lightning Source LLC
Chambersburg PA
CBHW060005300526
45794CB00003B/1089